MW00835360

Medical emergencies in Pediatric Dentistry

Vivek Mehta
Anupma Raheja Mehta

Medical emergencies in Pediatric Dentistry

LAP LAMBERT Academic Publishing

Impressum / Imprint

Bibliografische Information der Deutschen Nationalbibliothek: Die Deutsche Nationalbibliothek verzeichnet diese Publikation in der Deutschen Nationalbibliografie; detaillierte bibliografische Daten sind im Internet über http://dnb.d-nb.de abrufbar.

Alle in diesem Buch genannten Marken und Produktnamen unterliegen warenzeichen-, marken- oder patentrechtlichem Schutz bzw. sind Warenzeichen oder eingetragene Warenzeichen der jeweiligen Inhaber. Die Wiedergabe von Marken, Produktnamen, Gebrauchsnamen, Handelsnamen, Warenbezeichnungen u.s.w. in diesem Werk berechtigt auch ohne besondere Kennzeichnung nicht zu der Annahme, dass solche Namen im Sinne der Warenzeichen- und Markenschutzgesetzgebung als frei zu betrachten wären und daher von jedermann benutzt werden dürften.

Bibliographic information published by the Deutsche Nationalbibliothek: The Deutsche Nationalbibliothek lists this publication in the Deutsche Nationalbibliografie; detailed bibliographic data are available in the Internet at http://dnb.d-nb.de.

Any brand names and product names mentioned in this book are subject to trademark, brand or patent protection and are trademarks or registered trademarks of their respective holders. The use of brand names, product names, common names, trade names, product descriptions etc. even without a particular marking in this work is in no way to be construed to mean that such names may be regarded as unrestricted in respect of trademark and brand protection legislation and could thus be used by anyone.

Coverbild / Cover image: www.ingimage.com

Verlag / Publisher:
LAP LAMBERT Academic Publishing
ist ein Imprint der / is a trademark of
OmniScriptum GmbH & Co. KG
Heinrich-Böcking-Str. 6-8, 66121 Saarbrücken, Deutschland / Germany
Email: info@lap-publishing.com

Herstellung: siehe letzte Seite /
Printed at: see last page
ISBN: 978-3-659-61648-8

Zugl. / Approved by: Lucknow, King George Medical University, Diss., 2005

Copyright © 2014 OmniScriptum GmbH & Co. KG
Alle Rechte vorbehalten. / All rights reserved. Saarbrücken 2014

CONTENTS

INTRODUCTION

Life – Threatening emergencies can and do occur in the practice of pediatric dentistry. They can happen to anyone – a child patient, doctor, member of the office staff, or person who is merely accompanying a patient. Although the occurrence of these emergencies in dental office is infrequent, a number of factors existing today can increase the likelihood of such incidents including the therapeutic advances in the medical profession, the growing trend toward longer dental appointments and the increasing use and administration of drugs in dentistry.

Fortunately, other factors exist to minimize the development of life-threatening situations. These include a pretreatment physical evaluation of each patient, which consists of a medical history questionnaire, dialogue history, physical examination, and possible modifications in dental care to minimize medical risks.

In spite of the most meticulous protocols designed to prevent the development of life-threatening situations, emergencies still occur. The occurrence of a tragedy inside a dental office is not a surprising event given the stress many patients associate with dental care.

Although any medical emergency can develop in the dental office, some are seen more frequently than others. Most such situations are entirely stress induced (for example, pain, fear and anxiety) or involve pre-existing conditions that are exacerbated when patients are placed in stressful environments. Stress-induced situations include vasodepressor syncope and hyperventilation syndrome, whereas preexisting medical conditions that can be exacerbated by stress include most acute cardiovascular emergencies, asthma and seizures.

The effective management of pain and anxiety in the dental office is therefore essential in the prevention and minimization of potentially catastrophic situations.

Drug related adverse reactions comprise another category of life-threatening situations that occur more often than dentists expect. The most frequent are associated with local anesthetics and drugs most commonly used in dentistry. Psychogenic reactions, drug overdose and drug allergy are a few problems associated with the administration of local anesthetics. Most adverse responses are preventable. Therefore thorough knowledge of drug pharmacology and proper drug administration are critical in the prevention of drug-related complications.

In a survey conducted at the 2004 American Academy of Pediatric Dentistry (AAPD) "Pediatric Emergencies in the Dental Office" course the incidence of specific emergency situations reported were.

INCIDENCE OF SPECIFIC EMERGENCY SITUATIONS

	SITUATION	INCIDENTS
1.	Syncope (fainting)	75
2.	Hysteria	23
3.	Allergy, mild	22
4.	Seizures	13
5.	Hypoglycemia	9
7.	Aspiration	5
8.	Respiratory distress	4
9.	Bronchospasm	3
10.	Airway Obstruction	3
11	Allergy, Anaphylaxis	1
12.	Drug Overdose	1
13.	Cardiac arrest	1

Source
2004 AAPD, "Pediatric Emergencies in Dental Office"

PREVENTION OF MEDICAL EMERGENCIES:

A complete system of physical evaluation for all prospective dental patients can prevent approximately 90% of life-threatening situations. The remaining 10% (so-called sudden, unexpected deaths) occur in spite of all preventive efforts.

Preparation for an emergency diminishes the danger or possibility of morbidity and death. Prior knowledge of a patient's physical condition enables the doctor to incorporate modifications into the planned dental treatment.

The important components of physical evaluation should be known as they can lead to a significant reduction in the occurrence of acute medical emergencies when used properly.

GOALS OF PHYSICAL EVALUATION

1. Determine the patient's ability to physically tolerate the stress involved in the planned treatment.

2. Determine the patient's ability to psychologically tolerate the stress involved in the planned treatment.

3. Determine whether treatment modifications are required to enable the patient to better tolerate the stress involved in the planned treatment.

4. Determine whether the use of psycho sedation is warranted.

   a. Determine which sedation technique is most appropriate.

b. Determine whether contraindication exist to any of the drugs to be used in the planned treatment.

Physical Evaluation:

The term physical evaluation will be employed to discuss the steps involved in fulfilling the goals, which have been mentioned before.

It may consist of three components.

I. Medical history questionnaire.

II. Physical examination.

III. Dialogue history

With the information collected from these three steps, the doctor will be better able to:

1. Determine the physical and psychological status of the patient.

2. Seek medical consultation if indicated, and

3. Institute appropriate modifications in dental therapy if indicated.

(I) MEDICAL HISTORY QUESTIONNAIRE

The use of written, patient-completed medical history questionnaires is a moral and legal necessity in the practice of both medicine and dentistry.

A questionnaire provides the doctor with valuable information about the physical and psychological condition of the prospective patient.

Two basic types of Medical History questionnaires:

1. Short form
2. Long form

Short Form

Provides basic information concerning a patient's medical history and is ideally suited for the doctor with considerable clinical experience in physical evaluation.

Long Form

Provides a more detailed database concerning the physical condition of the prospective patient. It is used most often in teaching situations and represents an ideal instrument for teaching physical evaluation.

The ultimate value of the medical history questionnaire will rest on the ability of the doctor to interpret its meaning and to them elicit additional information through the physical examination and dialogue history.

(II)   PHYSICAL EXAMINATION

Physical examination provides much of the information. It consists of the following:

1.   Monitoring of vital signs

2.   Visual inspection of the patient

3.   Function tests as indicated.

4.   Auscultation of heart and lungs, and lab tests as indicated.

The primary value of the physical examination is that it provides the doctor with important information concerning the physical condition of the patient immediately before the start of treatment as contrasted with the questionnaire, which provides historical information. The patient should undergo this minimal physical evaluation during an initial visit to the office before the initiation of any form of treatment.

1. **Vital Signs:** There are 6 vital signs

   a) Blood pressure.

   b) Heart rate and rhythm (pulse)

   c) Respiratory rate

   d) Temperature

   e) Height

   f) Weight

2. **Visual Inspection of the Patient:** It may provide the doctor with valuable information concerning the medical status and the patient's level of apprehension towards dentistry. Observation of the patient's posture, body movements, speech, and skin can assist in a diagnosis of possibly significant disorders that may previously have gone undetected.

3. **Additional Evaluation Procedure:** After the completion of previous steps a follow-up with additional evaluation for specific medical disorders may on occasion be necessary. This examination may include auscultation of the heart and lungs, testing for urinary and blood glucose levels, retinal examination, function tests for cardio-respiratory status, electrocardiographic examination and blood chemistries. At present many of these tests are used in dental offices but do not represent the standard of care in dentistry.

(III) DIALOGUE HISTORY

On completion of gathering all of the information of doctor must sit down with the patient and attempt to determine the severity of any disorders and the potential risk represented by the patient during the planned treatment.

The process of discussion with the patient is termed the **Dialogue History** and it forms an integral part of patient evaluation. The doctor must use all available knowledge of the disease to accurately assess the degree of risk to the patient.

MEDICAL CONSULTATION

A number of steps are involved in a typical medical consultation. These are:

- ❖ Obtain the patient's dental and medical histories.
- ❖ Complete the physical examination including both oral and general examination.
- ❖ Provide a tentative treatment plan based on the patient's oral needs.
- ❖ Make a general systemic assessment.
- ❖ Consult the patient's physician when appropriate, via telephone and ask for additional information about the patient.
- ❖ Present your treatment plan briefly including medications to be used and the degree of stress anticipated.
- ❖ After consultation write a complete report of the conversation for records and obtain a written report from the physician if possible.

A dentist should not seek a medical consultation until the patient's dental and physical evaluations are completed. The dentist should be prepared to discuss fully with the patient's physician the proposed dental treatment plan and any anticipated problems.

One of the most important considerations in medical consultation is the determination of the patient's ability to tolerate in relative safety the stress involved in the proposed dental treatment.

The advice of the patient's regular physician should be carefully considered. Whenever doubt remains after a consultation a second opinion from a specialist in the specific area of concern should be sought.

After a satisfactory consultation the dentist should implement the steps to minimize the perceived risk to the patient. The dentist holds the final responsibility for the dental treatment plan and it's risks.

In most cases, medical consultation alters the dental plan minimally or not at all. Specific treatment modifications represent potentially important steps the dentist may undertake to decrease the patient's risk.

PREPARATION OF MEDICAL EMERGENCIES

The dental office staff must be fully prepared to assist in the recognition and management of any emergency situation that may develop. Unless all office personnel are capable of effectively managing those few serious emergencies that may develop during the practice lifetime of the doctor, those situations may well become office catastrophes.

GENERAL PREPARATION: Office Personnel

Training:

The most important factor in the preparation of a dental office for medical emergencies will be training all office personnel including non-chair side personnel in the recognition and management of these situations.

Training should include an annual refresher course in emergency medicine that provides a general review of all aspects of the subject such as seizures, chest pain and respiratory difficulty, rather than just a review of basic life support.

Most emergency situations occurring in dental practice will prove to be readily manageable through the use of basic life support. Drug therapy will usually be relegated to a secondary role Training in advanced cardiac life support is being advocated more and more today. It involves the following subjects: adjuncts for airway control and ventilation; monitoring and dysrhythmia recognition; defibrillation and synchronized cardio version; cardiovascular pharmacology, acid-base balance; venipuncture and resuscitation of infants, including the newborn.

Although not essential for all dental practitioners, the knowledge and ability to use these techniques in emergency situations is invaluable.

Team Management

With all office personnel trained in the recognition and management of life-threatening situations, if is possible for each person to maintain the life of a victim alone or as a member of a trained emergency team.

The emergency team consists of 2-3 members; each having a predefined role in the management of an emergency. The doctor leads the team and is responsible for directing the actions of all other team members.

Team member-1 **Doctor** who is with the victim or who first reaches the victim when the emergency situation is noticed. He initiates steps of Basic life support (Airway, Breathing, Circulation), as indicated by the physical assessment of the victim.

Member-2 will act as a "**Circulating Nurse**" or "**Circulating Assistant**". A chair side assistant working alongside the doctor will serve in this capacity if the patient is the victim.

Primary assignments for member 2 are to assist member 1 with basic life support, as required; to monitor the vital signs of the victim and to otherwise assist as needed, such as positioning the victim, loosening a collar or belt, or activating the EMS (Emergency Medical Services) system by dialing the appropriate telephone number.

The third member will be responsible for gathering up the emergency kit and portable oxygen. The person is also assigned to regularly check the supply of emergency drugs and oxygen to make certain they will be readily available when needed.

Emergency Practice Drills

In-office emergency drills are a means of maintaining an efficient emergency team in the absence of true emergency situations. On an irregular basis the doctor may stage a simulated life-threatening situation. All members of the team should be able to respond exactly as they must under emergency conditions.

Outside Medical Assistance

Although most dental office emergencies will be readily manageable by the emergency team, there may be occasion to call for outside medical assistance. Therefore emergency telephone numbers must be readily available and conspicuous at all telephones in the dental office. Telephone numbers to be included are:

- Local emergency medical services.
- A well-trained dental or medical professional
- Emergency ambulance services and
- A hospital emergency room.

EMERGENCY DRUG KITS

The dental office emergency kit should not be complicated.

However emergency kit is a simple organized collection of drugs and equipment found to be effective in managing life-threatening situations that indicate the administration of drugs.

First and foremost in the management of these situations will be the steps of basic life support. It is only after these steps have been taken that the doctor should consider the use of drugs. One exception is management of the acute allergic reactions, in which there is immediate respiratory embarrassment of circulatory collapse or both. In this situation treatment of choice will be the administration of epinephrine a soon s possible following the institution of basic support.

The following things should be remembered:

1. Drugs are NOT necessary for the proper management of most emergencies.

2. Primary management of all emergency situations is Basic Life Support. (BLS).

3. When in doubt, NEVER medicate.

The emergency kit is designed separately for pediatric patient, as pediatric doses are somewhat lower than adult doses.

Dosage forms of most drugs rarely differ, there being no dosage form specific for pediatric use with another form for the adult.

Naloxone, however is an exception being available in both adult and pediatric strengths.

Several items of emergency equipment should be available in both adult and pediatric sizes. Pediatric dentist must have a wider range of equipment available in both pediatric and adult sizes- than the doctor who does not treat younger patients.

EMERGENCY EQUIPMENT

Primary emergency equipment to be considered for the dental office includes:

1. Oxygen delivery system.

2. Suction and suction tips

3. Syringes for drug administration

4. Tourniquets

Secondary equipment include the following

5. Scalpel or cricothyrotomy needle.

6. Artificial Airways

7. Airway adjuncts.

Presence of various items of emergency equipment available does not of itself make the dental office any better equipped or the staff any more prepared to manage medical emergency situations.

Personnel expected to use this equipment must be well trained in the proper selection of patients and in the proper technique of use of these items.

Many of the emergency items commonly found in the dental office can prove to be useless or hazardous if employed improperly or on the wrong patient.

PRIMARY EMERGENCY EQUIPMENT

1. **Oxygen Delivery System**: An oxygen delivery system adaptable to the E cylinder of oxygen must allow for the delivery of possible pressure oxygen to the victim. Examples of this device include the positive pressure/demand value, and the reservoir bag on many inhalation units.

These devices should be fitted with clear face masks, which allow for the efficient delivery of oxygen or air to a patient while permitting the rescuer to visually inspect the mouth for the presence of foreign matter (vomits blood). Facemasks should be available in several sizes (child small adult and large adult). A portable self-inflating bag-mask valve device is a self-contained unit that may be easily transported to any site within the dental office. It is important because not all emergencies will occur within the dental office and it may be necessary to resuscitate the patient in other areas such as waiting room. A source of positive pressure oxygen or air must be available in these areas with both the devices the rescuer must be able to maintain both an airtight seal and a patent airway with one hand while using the other hand to ventilate the patient.

2. **Suction and Suction Tips**: An essential item is strong suction system and a variety of large diameter suction tips. The disposable saliva ejector is laterally inadequate in situations in which anything other than tiny objects must be evacuated from the mouth of a patient. Suction tips should be rounded to ensure that there is little hazard if it becomes necessary to suction the hypopharynx.

3. **Syringes for Drug Administration**: Plastic disposable syringes equipped with an 18 or a 21 gauge needle will be needed for drug administration 2 ml. syringe will be entirely adequate.

4. **Tourniquets**: It will be required if intravenous drug administration is contemplated. In addition three tourniques will be needed for management

of the patient in acute pulmonary edema. A sphygmomanometer (blood pressure cuff) may be employed as a tourniquet, as may a simple piece of latex tubing.

SECONDARY EMERGENCY EQUIPMENT

5.   **Scalpel or Cricothyrotomy Device**: As a final step in airway maintenance, if may become necessary to perform a cricothyrotomy. Therefore the emergency kit should contain a scalpel or a cricothyrotomy device.

6.   **Artificial Airways**: Plastic or rubber oropharyngeal or nasopharyngeal airways are used to assist in maintenance of a patent airway. They act by lifting the base of a tongue off to the posterior pharyngeal wall. They are used in causes where manual methods of maintaining an airway have proved ineffective.

Several sizes should always be available (i.e. child, small adult, normal adult) when oropharyngeal or nasopharyngeal airways are included in the emergency kit.

7.   **Airways Adjuncts**: Many devices are available to aid in the management of a patent airway. These include the

- S tube
- Esophageal obturator airway
- Endotracheal tube
- Laryngoscope
- Mc Grill intubation forceps

Training in the use of each item is absolutely essential.

ORGANIZING THE EMERGENCY KIT

A simple means of storing emergency drugs is in tackle box or plastic box with several compartments. Labels should be applied to cubicles storing each drug and should give the drugs generic name and brand name to avoid possible confusion during an emergency. Written records should be kept of the expiration date of each of the drugs in the emergency kit, and the drug should be replaced prior to its expiration date. Expired drugs as well as empty oxygen cylinders are ineffective in the management of any emergency situation. The emergency kit and equipment should be kept in a readily accessible area. The back of a storage closet is not the place for life-saving equipment.

COMMON MEDICAL EMERGENCIES and THEIR TREATMENT

1. SYNCOPE:

Etiology:

Syncope is a transient form of unconsciousness from which the patient can be roused. This is in contrast to coma, in which the patient is in a state of unconsciousness from which he cannot be roused. Women tend to faint more readily than men.

This tendency may be due to minor factors such as prolonged standing, high humid temperatures, long hours of work, lack of sleep, overheated poorly ventilated rooms, abrupt changes in altitude, fatiguing exertions, or hyperventilation. Pain, early6 pregnancy, blood loss and sharp blows also induce fainting, as can many drugs.

Drugs associated with syncope are those that lower blood pressure, insulin (overdose), phenacetin, diuretics, and procaine.

Physiology:

It is due to impaired cerebral metabolism, which is caused by a brief derivation of oxygen and glucose to the brain. This phenomenon occurs as a results of:

1. A transient decrease in cardiac output

2. A decrease in arterial pressure.

3. A change in blood composition, usually a decrease in oxygen and glucose in the blood delivered to the brain.

Prevention

The proper assessment of the patient is the single most important factor. A medical history of any present illness, especially of a respiratory or cardiac nature and also of previous serious illnesses must be taken. Current and past drug therapy esp. with antihypertensive, diuretics, tranquilizers, MAO inhibitors, antibiotics, insulin, thyroid, steroids and anticoagulants should be carefully noted.

Allergic tendencies and the patient's weight are also important factors to be aware of before commencing treatment under local anesthesia, sedatives or G.A. Drug therapy is effective, orally or intravenously, with dramatic results in patient comfort and acceptance of dental procedures.

II. RESPIRATORY DIFFICULTY

General Considerations: Difficulty in breathing can be a most disconcerting problem for a patient who is conscious yet unable to breathe normally. Because the patient usually remains conscious throughout the episode of respiratory difficulty, the psychological aspects of patient management are important.

Predisposing Factors: The list of potential causes of respiratory difficulty is as follows:

S.No.	Cause	Frequency
1.	Hyperventilation syndrome	Most common
2.	Vasodepressor Syncope	Most common
3.	Asthma	Common
4.	Heart failure	Common
5.	Hypoglycemia	Common
6.	Overdose reaction	Less Common
7.	Acute myocardial infarction	Rare
8.	Anaphylaxis	Rare
9.	Angio neurotic edema	Rare
10.	Cerebrovascular accident	Rare
11.	Epilepsy	Rare
12.	Hyperglycemic reaction	Rare

The hyperventilation syndrome and vasodepressor syncope which represent the most commonly encountered emergency situations in dentistry are almost exclusively precipitated by psychological stress.

Psychological stress in dentistry is the primary factor in the intensification of preexisting medical disorders.

Although hyperventilation and vasodepressor syncope are rarely causes of respiratory difficulty in pediatric patients, children with asthma may exhibit acute episodes of bronchospasm in stressful situations.

Prevention: Adequate pretreatment medical and dental evaluation of the prospective dental patient can often prevent respiratory difficulty. Once aware of medical disorders that may lead to these problems the doctor can modify patient management to minimize the exacerbation of these conditions. When anxiety is a major factor, psycho sedative procedures and stress-reduction techniques can be employed.

Clinical Manifestations: They vary according to the degree of breathing difficulty. In most cases the patient remains conscious throughout the episode.

The sounds associated with distressed breathing and the clinical symptoms vary with the cause of the problem.

Pathophysiology: Various parts of the respiratory system are involved in the different syndromes producing respiratory difficulty.

Asthma: Bronchioles are the primary site of the disorder. Bronchi become highly reactive and demonstrate significant smooth muscle activity in response to various substances.

21

Heart Failure: Respiratory difficulty is usually the first sign and symptom noted. It is produced by chronic over utilization of the oxygen in the blood and an inability of the lungs to fully oxygenate blood. It is related to pulmonary engorgement with exudation of fluid into alveolar air sacs. This excess fluid prevents portions of the lung from participating in the ventilator process producing many of the signs and symptoms associated with heart failure.

Hyper Ventilation Syndrome: is a generalized problem. The primary site is in mind of the patient and its clinical signs and symptoms are due to alteration in the clinical makeup of the blood. An excessive amount of CO_2 is eliminated through rapid breathing leading to respiratory alkalosis.

This in turn produces many of the clinical signs and symptoms of hyperventilation. If successfully managed, this syndrome produces no residual effects

Acute Lower Airway Obstruction: is a life-threatening situation in which a foreign object becomes occluded in the respiratory tract. The level at which this object occludes the airway determines the severity of the situation and to some degree the manner in which it may be managed. If an object enters either of the bronchi the situation is dangerous but not life threatening.

It usually enters right mainstream bronchus because of the angle at which this branches off of the trachea.

Management of Respiratory Difficulty:

1.   Recognition of respiratory difficulty

- Sounds (wheezing, cough)

- Abnormal rate and/or depth respiration

2   Termination of dental procedure

3.   Position patient, implement basic life support.

- Unconscious-supine position.

- Conscious-Upright position usually preferred by patient

4.   Monitor vital signs.

- Blood pressure, heart rate (pulse); respiratory rate

5.   Symptomatic management of patient.

6.   Definitive Management of respiratory difficulty.

Sequences for removing airway obstruction.

III.   ALTERED CONSCIOUSNESS:

A number of systemic medical conditions may manifest themselves clinically as alterations in the victim's state of consciousness.

Causes of Altered Consciousness:

S.No.	Cause	Frequency
1.	Drug overdose (alcohol, insulin, barbiturates)	Most Common
2.	Hyperventilation syndrome	Common
3.	Hypoglycemia	Common
4.	Hyperglycemia	Less Common
5.	Cerebrovascular accident, transient ischemic attack	Less Common
6.	Hyperthyroidism	Rare
7.	Hypothyroidism	Rare

Altered consciousness may be the first clinical sign of a serious medical problem that requires immediate and intensive therapy to maintain the victims life.

It is important therefore that the doctor be aware of a patient medical background in order to recognize the developing medical problem when it arises and to manage any emergency that may develop at a later time.

Predisposing Factors: The most common cause is the ingestion or administration of drugs with the increasing use of psycho-sedation in dental practice, we are likely to encounter these agents to patients. Proper use of these drugs minimizes these incidents.

The hyperventilation syndrome is the most common non-drug cause of altered consciousness. Acute anxiety is the precipitating factor in almost all instances of hyperventilation. It is seen primarily in younger patients (<40 years).

Other systemic situations include-diabetes mellitus, cerebrovascular ischemia and infarction and thyroid gland dysfunction.

❖ Diabetes mellitus and its associated acute clinical complications hypoglycemia and hyperglycemia are commonly encountered in dental patients. Inadequate medical management of the disease and the presence of stress may rapidly lead to an altered state of consciousness and possibility to the loss of episodes of hypoglycemia in certain circumstances.

❖ Cerebrovascular ischemia and infarction (stroke) are other less common but potentially more serious causes of altered consciousness. Proper management of the post cerebrovascular accident patient greatly reduces the chance of a second incident precipitated by dental therapy.

❖ Thyroid gland dysfunction also results in state of altered consciousness. Although acute clinical complications from thyroid hypofunction or hyperfunction are rare in dental situations the doctor must be aware of the presence of thyroid gland dysfunction and be able to recognize signs and symptoms of thyroid complications.

There is greatly increased incidence of cardiovascular disease in these persons.

In all of these situations increased stress decreases the patient's ability to withstand dental therapy without disease-related complications.

Prevention: Recognition of unusually high levels of apprehension in a prospective dental patient minimizes the occurrence of vasodepressor syncope and the hyperventilation syndrome. Proper use of psycho sedative techniques prevent treatment related drug overdose.

In other situations prior awareness of patient's medical condition allows the doctor to modify the proposed therapy to minimize the risk to patient. The health questionnaire, physical examination and recording of vital signs are valuable in the proper assessment of this patient.

Clinical Manifestations: They include the cold, wet appearance mental confusion and bizarre behavior of the hypoglycemic patient contrast with the hot, dry, florid appearance of the hyperglycemic diabetic patient. The presence of "**acetone breath**" further aids in the clinical recognition of hyperglycemia.

Cerebro-vascular accident (stroke) may occur with a sudden onset of unconsciousness or a more gradual onset of symptoms related to CNS dysfunction

These symptoms may include variable degree of derangement of speech, thought, motion, sensation or vision. The patient may be alert and may demonstrate degrees of alteration of consciousness ranging from headache, dizziness and drowsiness to mental confusion.

Hypothyroidism if untreated may cause symptoms of weakness, fatique, lethargy and slow speech.

Untreated hyperthyroidism causes restlessness, nervousness, irritability and degrees of motor in coordination ranging from a fine milk tremulousness to gross tremor.

MANAGEMENT

Step -1   Recognition of altered consciousness

        Skin   Cold and wet

                    Hot and dry

                    Hot with excessive sweating

                    Cold and dry

        Breath   "Acetone" breath

        Headache, dizziness, confusion

Step-2   Terminate dental procedure

Step-3 Position patient

Conscious upright position usually preferred by patient.

Unconscious supine position.

If CVA is considered and elevated blood pressure is present, head and thorax should be elevated slightly.

Step-4   Basic Life support

Step-5   Monitor vital signs

                Blood pressure, heart rate (pulse), respiratory rate and temperature

Step-6   Management of signs and symptoms

Step-7   Definitive management

DRUG RELATED EMRGENCIES

The administration of drugs has become common place within the practice of dentistry. Local anesthetic agents, analgesics, antibiotics and antianxiety drugs are the four categories of drug which constitute the majority of drugs used in the practice of dentistry.

Indiscriminate use of drugs has become one of the major causes of the great increase in the number of serious incidents of drug-related life threatening in emergencies that are being reported. Most drug-related emergency situations are classified as one aspect of iatrogenic disease, a category that encompasses an entire spectrum of adverse effects produced unintentionally by physicians or dentists during the management of their patients.

- **Toxicology**: is defined as the study of the harmful effects of chemicals on biologic systems. Some general principles of toxicology must be kept in mind.

1. No drug ever exerts a single action.
2. No clinically useful drug is entirely devoid of toxicity.
3. Potential toxicity of a drug rests in the hands of the user.

- Prevention: Drug use within the practice of dentistry is absolutely essential for the safe and proper management of many dental patients. Therefore it is important for the doctor to become familiar with the pharmacologic properties of all drugs used in dental practice.

- All drugs are capable of producing harm if handled improperly and conversely and drug may be handled safety if proper precautions are observed. The potential toxicity of a drug rests in the hands of the user. A second factor in the safe use of drugs is consideration of the patient to whom the drug will be administered. Individuals may react differently to the some stimulus; patients therefore vary marked in their reactions to drugs.

CLASSIFICATION

The classification proposed by Pallasch represents a simplified approach to the problem of classifying adverse drug reactions.

1. Toxicity resulting from direct extension of pharmacologic effects.

    i.   Side effects

    ii.   Abnormal dosage (cover dosage)

    iii.   Local toxic effects.

2. Toxicity resulting from altered recipient (patient)

- Present of pathology
- Emotional disturbances
- Genetic aberrations (idiosyncrasy)
- Teratogenicity
- Drug-drug interactions.

3. Toxicity resulting from drug allergy.

There are normally three situations that are of immediate importance to the dental practitioner.

Over dose, allergy and Idiosyncrasy

Over Dose Reaction: Overdose reaction refers to symptoms resulting from an absolute or relative over administration of a drug that produces elevated blood levels of the agent. Clinical manifestations of overdose are related to a direct expansion of the normal pharmacologic actions of the agent.

In therapeutic doses barbiturates for example produce mild depression of the central nervous system, which results in sedation or hypnosis (desired effects). Barbiturate overdose produces a more profound depression of the CNS with possible respiratory and cardiovascular depression.

Local anesthetics are also CNS depressants. When administered properly and therapeutic doses little or no evidence of CNS depression is evident, however with increased blood levels signs and symptoms of selective CNS depression are noted:

Allergy: It may be defined as a hypersensitive state acquired through exposure to a particular allergen, re exposure to which bring about a heightened capacity to react. Clinically allergy expresses itself as drug fever, angioedema, urticaria, dermatitis, depression of the blood forming organs, photosensitivity and anaphylaxis.

Certain drugs are more likely to cause allergic reactions then others and allergic reaction is possible with any substance.

In contrast to the overdose reaction in which clinical manifestations are related directly to the pharmacologic properties, allergic reaction is always produced by exaggerated response to the immune system of the body.

The degree of this response determines the acuteness of the reaction.

Idiosyncratic Reaction: Adverse Drug reactions that cannot be explained by any known pharmacologic or biochemical mechanism.

An example of idiosyncratic reaction is CNS stimulation (excitation, agitation) produced followed the administration of a known CNS depressant agents as a barbiturate. Idiosyncratic reactions span an extremely wide range of clinical expression.

It is impossible to predict which person will experience the reactions or the nature of the resulting idiosyncratic reactions.

Management: Because of the unpredictability of the nature and occurrence of idiosyncratic reactions, their management is symptomatic. Of primary concern in the management of these situations are the essentials of basic life support: Maintenance of the airway, ventilation and circulation. Prevention of injury and airway management are the primary considerations.

DENTAL PATIENT WITH CONVULSIVE DISORDERS

A convulsion by a patient in a dental office can be frightening and disruptive.

A Convulsion is a paroxysmal disorder of the brain characterized by focal or generalized inappropriate uncontrolled discharges from neurons resulting in multiple impairments of neurologic functioning.

A convulsion is synonymous with seizures fits or epileptic attacks. The clinical expression of a convulsion disorder is varied. Some attacks are preceded by an aura which is often quite specific for a given patient but is quite variable from patient to patient. The aura may be a simple psychic or somatic feeling, a more dramatic focal or generalized sensory disturbance, or a rather complex auditory, visual or gustatory hallucination. Not all auras are followed by an overt convulsion.

The convulsion varies considerably from patient to patient. At one end of the spectrum is a mild alteration of mental functioning without loss of consciousness with some mild involuntary motor activity such as rapid eye blinking or alteration of muscle tone. At the other end is the sudden loss of consciousness with the immediate onset of involuntary tonic and/or clonic, focal or generalized motor activity perhaps with impairment of breathing, bluish discoloration, foaming at the mouth, tongue biting and incontinence of bowels and/or bladder.

Many convulsions are followed by a postictal state characterized by a few moments of mental convulsion or perhaps a more dramatic profound deep sleep lasting several hours followed by gradual awakening associated with severe headache and muscle soreness .

The clinical manifestations may vary with the patient's age. Most children have convulsions in which clinical manifestations would be a simple kinetic convulsion or drop attack, in which the patient will suddenly losses all motor tone, resulting in potentially injurious fall which may or may not be associated with impairment of consciousness.

They are also prone to petit mal convulsion characterized by the sudden impairment of consciousness with relatively preserved general motor tone and associated with frequent rapid eye movements, all lasting for seconds and followed by an immediate return to the preconvulsive state of functioning.

The amount of provocation required to induce convulsive activity is referred to as the "Convulsive threshold" which varies amongst the individual's. High fever can induce such activity particularly in children.

Physicians vary somewhat in their evaluation of a patient who presents with convulsion.

Basic to most investigations are determination of B.P., listening for evidence of carotid artery insufficiency, listening for evidence of valvular heart disease and looking for evidence of systemic illness such as major metabolic disorders, anemia or malignancy.

Laboratory investigations consist of CBC, fasting and/or 2 hour post-prandial blood sugar, BUN, calcium and magnesium. A electroencephalogram and computerized axial tomography (CAT) of the brain are integral parts of the evaluation.

Most convulsions can be completely controlled or significantly influenced with a single medication or a combination of medications- Barbiturates, Hydantoins, oxazolidinediones, succinimides.

The chronic use of anticonvulsant medications is at times complicated by several problems including bone marrow suppression and hepatotoxicity. From a dental point of view bone marrow suppression might be a factor in a dental patient's ability to combat actual or anticipated infection or the ability to form an appropriate blood clot. Also of dental significance is the tendency of dilantin to promote gingival hyperplasia.

If a convulsion occurs in a dental office it is important to note the five of onset as most convulsions in a given patient tend to last a predictable period to time that is unique to the patient.

During the actual convulsion the patient should be placed on the floor and rolled to either side so that if emesis occurs there is a decreased chance of aspiration.

It is not necessary to restrain flailing motor movements other than to protect the patient from self-injury.

If possible a soft object should be placed between the teeth taking special care not to wedge the tongue between that object and the teeth.

If a convulsion lasts longer than usual for a given patient and attending physician has not been contacted, intravenous administration of Valium 5 to 10 mg or Amytal 125 mg over 3-5 minutes would be an appropriate step to stop the convulsion assuming there has not been a previous poor or adverse response to such treatments.

Special care is necessary to note any respiratory distress that would dictate discontinuation of the medication.

The patient should be advised to contact the treating physician so that additional investigation or alteration of medication can be carried out.

With teamwork between the patient, dentist and physician, the chance of a convulsion in the dental office can be minimized.

CARDIAC ARREST AND CARDIOPULMONARY RESUSCITATION

Angina pectoris, myocardial infarction, and heart failure are three clinical manifestations of arteriosclerosis of the coronary arteries. Associated with each of these clinical situations in the possible development of acute complications, among these are cardiac arrest or sudden death. Cardiac arrest may also occur as a clinical entity in the absence of other cardiovascular manifestations.

Ventricular fibrillation is the major cause of death from ischemic heart disease. It most often occurs within the first 2 hours following the onset of clinical symptoms of coronary artery disease.

Ventricular fibrillation is often reversible if adequate oxygenation of the myocardium is maintained until defibrillation is successfully carried out. Adequate circulation of the steps of basic life support (BLS).

DISORDERS ASSOCIATED WITH CARDIOPULMONARY ARREST

- Respiratory Failure:
- Hypoxemia-any cause.
- Airway obstruction foreign body croup, epiglottitis.
- Lung dysfunction-Pneumonia, asthma, pneumothorax.

Circulatory failure:

Hypovolemic-dehydration, hemorrhage

Septic-Neisseria meningitides, Hemophilus influenza

Metabolic:

- Acidosis, electrolyte abnormalities

Central Nervous System:

- Apnea, increased intracranial pressure (trauma, mass lesions, infection)

If BLS is not begun immediately the victims brain is hypoxic for a longer period to time before circulation of oxygenated blood is restored. Permanent damage (biologic death) to neuronal tissues is more severe and the victims chance of having a level of neurologic activity close to the pre-arrest level is decreased.

Basic life support consists of airway maintenance artificial ventilation and external chest compression of the victim so that a continuous support of oxygenated blood is delivered to the brain and heart thereby preventing non reversible (biologic) death.

SUMMARY FOR PEDIATRIC BASIC LIFE SUPPORT

	INFANT	CHILD
Airway	Head-tilt/chin- lift Jaw-thrust	Head-tilt/chin- lift Jaw-thrust
Breathing Initial Rate	Two breaths 20 breaths/min	Two breaths 15 breaths/min
Circulation Pulse check Compression technique Depth Compression/ ventilation Ratio	Brachial/Femoral Lower 1/3 of sternum With 2-3 fingers 0.5-1.0 inch 5:1 (Pause for ventilation)	Carotid Lower 1/3 of sternum With heel of hand 1.0-1.5 inch 5:1 (Pause for ventilation)
Foreign body in Airway	Back blows/ chest thrust	Heimlich Maneuver

CHILD RESUSCITATION

For the purpose of basic life support technique the child is a person between the ages of 1 and 8 years.

Basic procedures for resuscitation of the child are similar to adult and infant.

The shake and shout maneuver is employed to determine lack of responsiveness, help is called for, and the patient is placed in the supine position.

The airway of the child is maintained by head tilt-chin lift and is then assessed for the presence of spontaneous respiratory efforts. If absent two full ventilation are provided.

The carotid pulse is assessed for 5 to 10 seconds and if absent the EMS system is activated and external chest compressions are begum.

The sternum is compressed 1 to 1½ inches (2.5 to 3.8 cm) at a ratio of 5 compressions to 1 ventilation, at a rate of 80 to 100 compressions per minute (5 every 3 to 4 seconds)

After 10 cycles (60 to 87 seconds) and periodically thereafter the patient should be evaluated for the return of spontaneous pulse and/or respiration.

SURGICAL AND OPERATIVE EMERGENCIES:

Surgical emergencies and complications are encountered in every dental practice that includes surgical procedures in its scope. No dentist should include surgery in his practice unless he is prepared to cope with emergencies and complications when they arise and unless he possesses the knowledge and skill to manage the problems successfully.

- Before undertaking and surgical procedure a thorough pre-operative evaluation of the patient should be made.

- The evaluation should include a careful history, a thorough clinical examination, adequate roentgenograms, and any necessary laboratory procedures.

- An excellent example of the importance of the preoperative evaluation is the serious bleeding problem that arises when extractions are preformed on an unprepared hemophiliac.

- To prevent emergencies and complications no surgical procedure should be performed on the teeth or supporting structures until adequate roentgenograms are available. Procedures carried out without roentgenograms may result in fractured roots, fractured alveolar process, involvement of maxillary sinus, nerve injury etc.

- Emergencies will be minimized if a well thought out, well regulated surgical plan is formulated before the procedure is started.

- Adherence to sound surgical principles at time of surgery is essential to reduce further risk of emergencies.

The principles include: adequate exposure of the operative field, hemostasis, adequate but conservative removal of bone when indicated, use of controlled force, careful debridement and closure of the wound and the conservative manipulation of tissue at all times.

It is impossible to cover all the emergencies and complications of exodontias and oral surgery therefore more common surgical emergencies seen in a busy dental practice will be covered.

ACUTE INFECTIONS

Acutely infected tooth is one of the most commonly encountered surgical emergencies. It is manifested by a swollen face, an elevated temperature and varying degrees of pain. Patient has spent one or more sleepless nights, is dehydrated and may have eaten little. Local examination reveals extremely tender, sore, loose tooth.

There may or may not be fluctuation in the soft tissues signifying localization of the infectious process.

Most oral surgeons now believe that the conservative treatment of the acutely infected tooth is no longer indicated and that immediate extraction of the involved tooth is the procedure of choice. By using adequate pre and postoperative antibiotic therapy and extracting the offending tooth by an atraumatic surgical procedure. Under general or regional block anesthesia, early resolution of the infectious process may be expected.

Removal of the tooth produces immediate relief from pain and usually results in reduction of swelling by the following day with complete resolution of the supportive process without untoward complications.

Immediate extraction satisfies the basic surgical principle of "removal of the cause", and permits drainage of the original focus through the socket. Any collection of pus in the soft tissue may be evacuated at the same time by adequate incision and drainage.

PERICORONAL INFECTIONS

It is another surgical emergency frequently encountered. It usually occurs in young people during the eruption process of the third molars with the mandibular teeth being the most frequent offenders. The oral mucosa is broken by a cusp of the erupting tooth. This causes development of infection under and about the pericoronal flap. The region is hot, moist, dark and contains decomposed food products in which rapid growth of bacteria may occur. This infectious process develops rapidly and often spreads to contiguous structures resulting in trismus, pain, sore throat, swelling and difficulty in swallowing. At times it produces hyperpyrexia, chills, rapid pulse and general malaise.

Some feel that treatment should include the immediate removal of the involved tooth, others believe that surgery is almost never indicated in the initial treatment of this infectious condition.

The correct answer lies midway between these two extremes and depends upon a thorough evaluation of each case. If the infectious process is more or less limited to the immediate surrounding soft tissue and if the offending tooth is so situated that its removal could be accomplished by a simple surgical procedure with minimal trauma to the surrounding soft tissue then the immediate removal of the tooth with indicated supportive measures consisting of antibiotics and strong analgesics, would be the treatment of choice.

If the infectious process is diffuse and the causative tooth is in a position that its removal would require a complicated prolonged procedure necessitating the formation of soft tissue flaps and removal of osseous structures and sectioning the tooth, it would be best to treat the pericoronal infection until its resolves before undertaking removal of the tooth.

In treatment of the pericoronal infection before extraction, drainage and irrigation of the pericoronal pocket are the important factors. This is done by passing a blunt instrument under the flap and displacing the flap upward. This periods adequate escape of a small amount of purulent discharge form the pocket. It this does not permit adequate drainage, the mucosa overlying the tooth should be incised. The area is then irrigated with normal saline using a 100 cc syringe with a blunt, curved, 13 gauge needle. This mechanical lavage washes out debris and facilitates drainage of the area. An iodoform gauze or a rubber drain may be placed under the flap and extended back into the pericoronal pocket as it prevents further accumulation of debris and infectious material in the pocket and allows for continuous drainage.

Following treatment of the pericoronal infection it should be determined if the maxillary 3rd molar is impinging on the swollen tissue surrounding the mandibular tooth. If this occurs it is good judgment to extract the maxillary tooth during the first visit.

Following these procedures the patient should be maintained on antibiotic therapy and strong analgesics and seen daily for further irrigation and treatment

ALVEOLAR OSTEITIS

It is a painful postoperative condition produced by disintegration of the clot in a tooth socket. This is a painful condition, which is the result of a surgical procedure, and correct management is important.

This condition is due to a loss of the blood clot which acts as a bandage toprotect the underlying osseous tissue. With loss of the clot, nerve endings in the bone become exposed to the oral cavity resulting in pain. Thus any condition interfering with formation and maintenance of a healthy clot in the socket can be incriminated as causing the condition.

Prevention: Insertion of antibiotic or chemotherapeutic cones in the socket, perforating the cortical bone surrounding the socket to insure a more adequate blood supply, general supportive care, vitamin, therapy systemic antibiotic therapy etc. are the measures utilized.

Treatment: It is directed towards relief of pain and stimulation of normal repair of the extraction would.

For the most part a dressing containing an obtundant to relieve the pain and an antiseptic to combat any infection that may be present is used.

Before applying the dressing the socket should be cleansed of all remaining disintegrated clot soothe medication may come in direct contact with the bone. This is done by irrigation or by light curettage.

The bone should then be dried and a dressing containing one of the many analgesics and antiseptic drugs in a liquid or paste form should be applied. The dressing should give relief from pain within a few minutes and keep the patient comfortable for longer than 24 hours, a dry socket should not be dressed every day because the manipulation of the socket will interfere with the proliferation of repair tissues and prolong the recovery period.

One dressing,which meets the criteria of having a prolonged effect and require changing only every 2nd, 3rd or 4th day.

- Eugenol   46%
- Balsam Peru   46%
- Chlorobutanol   04%
- Benzocaine   04%

The dressing should be placed on iodoform or plain gauze and applied loosely in the socket, covering all the exposed bone.

Curettage of the exposed bone has been advocated as a means of stimulating bleeding and causing a new blood clot to form in the socket.

THERMAL BURNS

Heated instruments utilized in the mouth produce painful burns when allowed to come in contact with the mucosa. Overheated hand pieces or rotating instruments coming in contact with the skin or mucosa are other causes of thermal burns.

Such wounds seldom require treatment. Suturing is not indicated, and the wound usually will heal rapidly by secondary intention.

If pain is a problem, it may be relieved by covering the wound with a protective medicament such as Bucrylate, Orabase or Tincture of benzoin.

When utilizing hot instruments or rotating instruments that may become overheated, the operator should exert every precaution to keep them from contacting the skin to prevent soft tissue would.

AVULSION

A true dental emergency exists with complete avulsion of the tooth from the alveolar segment. The prognosis of the pulp and periodontal tissue is directly related to the proper diagnosis and to the action taken at the scene of the accident, usually not by dentally trained individuals. The most frequently involved teeth are the maxillary central incisors, the injury usually occurring between the ages of 7 and 10 when the permanents incisors are erupting. According to Andreasen (1981), the loosely structured periodontal ligaments and resilient alveolar bone surrounding erupting teeth favour avulsion over other injuries.

The goal of replantation of teeth following traumatic avulsion is to maintain the viability to the cells of the pulp and periodontal ligament to assist reattachment and avoid posttraumatic complications of root resorption. The success of replantation is inversely related to the length of time the tooth is out of the socket. Andreasen and Hjorting Hanson (1981) observed that after a period of 2 or more years 90% of teeth replanted less than 30 minutes after avulsion exhibited no discernible root resorption. Conversely, root resorption was seen in 95% of the teeth with an extraoral period of greater than 2 hours. Root resorption involves loss of the root structure secondary to the inflammatory response associated with loss of pulpal and periodontal ligament vitality and rapid loss of the replanted tooth.

Even short periods of root surface drying may have adverse effects on the periodontal ligament. Because time is critical, replantation at the site of injury has the best prognosis. Ambulance attendants or supervising adults should be instructed to place the tooth so that it is even with the neighbouring teeth and looks like the same tooth on the opposite side of the involved jaw. After replantation the tooth should be held in place with light pressure from a finger (rather than biting on a washcloth, which may force the tooth laterally) en route to the office or clinic. If the tooth cannot be replaced it should be stored in the buccal vestibule of the cheek or under the tongue of the patient unless because of the extent of injury or the age and cooperation of the child there is a concern of aspiration or swallowing of the tooth. If there are such problems the tooth can be stored in the mouth of the supervising adult for transportation without adverse consequences. If neither option is a available the tooth can be stored in milk or saline (one teaspoon of salt added to 8 ounces of water or saliva-socked towel). Storage in tap water has been documented to have adverse affects on periodontal healing. The tooth should never be allowed to dry.

Upon arrival at the Emergency Department the teeth and traumatized tissue should be inspected to determine if the tooth is primary. The tooth root should be evaluated for evidence of resorption or radiograph taken of the alveolar bone to locate the succedaneous tooth. Avulsed primary teeth should not be replanted.

The avulsed tooth should not be replanted if there is advanced periodontal disease a condition seldom seen in children to teenagers. There should not be extensive damage to the socket site and the extra oral period must be less than 2 hours. Gingival lacerations should be sutured and a tetanus booster should be given if more than 5 years have passed since the last tetanus immunization.

Follow up examinations with radiographic and vitality evaluations must be done to avoid loss of the tooth. Patients with injured teeth should be followed by a family dentist responsible for continued care.

DENTOALVEOLAR FRACTURES

Dentoalveolar fractures and involved tooth trauma with maxillary or mandibular fractures require evaluation and treatment by an oral and maxillofacial surgeon. Alveolar socket fractures are usually associated with luxation injuries. There is usually mobility to the underlying bone with the involved teeth and evidence of contusion or laceration of the gingival. Reduction of the fracture involves simultaneous digital pressure on the crown and along the fracture site with or without local anesthesia. After reduction of the fracture the occlusion should be checked with the involved teeth splinted and removed from occlusal movement. Gingival lacerations should be sutured. Alveolar process fractures in young children may not need to be reduced and the child should be maintained on a soft diet for 2 weeks.

Follow Up Care

A child with possible traumatic injury to the teeth or supporting structures should see a dentist for periodic follow up evaluations. Ideally this family or pediatric dentist has been trained to manage trauma to the pediatric dentition, which often requires different technique than are used for permanent dentition. Long term follow up is essential especially in patients with blunt trauma to the teeth or lips as degeneration of the pulpal tissue, pulpal necrosis or resorption of the dentin or cementum of the tooth may not be detected for several months following trauma.

Facila Infections

The teeth are frequently the sources of infection, facial swelling, and pain in the pediatric population. Dental caries is the most common infectious disease that affects both the primary and the permanent dentition. The breakdown of the enamel and dentinal layers of the tooth may eventually lead to bacterial invasion of the pulpal tissues. The pulp contains the blood and nervous supply to the tooth within the restrictive pulp chamber. The pulp tissue will react to the bacterial invasion by a typical inflammatory response, which usually is quite painful to the patient due to the constructive nature of the pulp within the tooth and the small apical foramina in the tooth. If the infection is allowed to progress, the pulp may become abscessed and breakdown outside the tooth with facial swelling. Children have a tendency to become quickly dehydrated with tooth pain and this compounds the management since they may quickly become systemically ill.

PSYCHOSOCIAL EMERGENCIES

Domestic violence is an ever increasing problem in modern day society and includes abuse directed against children.

Dentists are frequently the first health professionals to render treatment to an abused patient.

Child Abuse is the single diagnostic term used to describe a range of behaviours from somewhat harsh discipline to intentional repetitive torture.

Abuse can be subdivided into 4 broad categories:

1. Physical Abuse
2. Sexual Abuse
3. Neglect
4. Emotional Abuse

Each form of abuse has individual characteristics of family dynamics, clinical manifestations and management.

Public law defines "**Child Abuse and Neglect**" as "the physical and mental injury, sexual abuse, negligent treatment or maltreatment of a child under the age of eighteen by a person who is responsible for the childs welfare under circumstances which indicate that the child's health or welfare is harmed or threatened thereby".

An abused child includes any child who is the victim of sexual activity who is endangered or who exhibits evidence of any physical or mental injury or death acquired other than by accidental means or any injury or death which is at variance with the history given of it. The child may also be considered abused if, because of the acts or omissions of his or her parents, guardian, or custodian the child suffers physical or mental injury that harm or threatens to harm the child's health or welfare.

A neglected child is one who is abandoned, who lacks proper parental care because of the faults or habits of his or her caretakers, or whose parent's guardians or custodians neglect or refuse to provide proper or necessary subsistence, education, medical or surgical care or treatment, or any special care made necessary by his or her mental condition.

The National Center for Child Abuse and neglect has defined sexual abuse as "Contacts or interactions between a child and an adult when the child is being used for the sexual stimulation of the perpetrator or another person".

Sexual abuse may also be committed by person under the age of 18 when the person is significantly older than the victim or is in a position of power or control over the victim.

The distinction between sexual abuse and sexual assault may be drawn according to the relationship between the aggressor and the child. Thus, sexual contacts between a child and a parent, a baby-sitter, a teacher or any other person acting as caretaker is abuse, but the same contacts made by a person who is not a care-taker are termed sexual assault.

Sexually transmitted diseases and their probability of being caused by child sexual abuse.

Always	Usually	Possibly
• Neisseria gonorrhea • Syphilis	• Herpes simplex • Chlamydia trachomatis • Trichomoniasis	• Condylomata • Scabies • Pediculosis • Gardnerella Vaginalis

Early recognition with timely referrals to appropriate agencies can possibly help prevent more significant injuries and even death from occurring in abused patients.

EMERGENCY DRUGS

Two categories of emergency drugs will be described:

1. Injectable drugs.
2. Non-Injectable drugs.

These drug categories will be further divided into two additional groups.

1. Primary drugs-items that can be included but are not absolutely essential.

Several items of emergency equipment should be available in both adult and pediatric sizes especially in dental offices in which many children are treated. These items included the full-face mark and oropharyngeal and nasopharyngeal airways. The pedodontist must have a wider range of equipment and drugs available.

Injectable Drugs: There are twelve main drugs which make up the list of injectable drugs considered for inclusion in the dental office emergency kit. They should be considered essential (primary) drugs.

    a. Epinephrine (for management of acute allergic reactions.
    b. Anti histamine
    c. Anti convulsant
    d. Narcotic antagonist

Non essential (secondary) drugs are:
Non essential (secondary) drugs are

    e. Analgesic
    f. Vasopressor
    g. Antihypoglycemic

A third category of injectable drugs is included for doctors trained in ACLS (Advanced Cardiac Life Support). ACLS training is especially valuable for doctors employing parenteral sedation or general anesthetic techniques in their dental offices.

The drugs in the ACLS category are:

1.   Sodium bicarbonate

2.   Calcium chloride

3.   Lidocaine (cardiac)

4.   Atropine

Ideal technique of emergency drug administration will be the Intravenous (IV) technique. Onset of action is rapid and the drug effect is most reliable using this route of administration. Emergency medications may be administered intramuscularly (IM) into various sites, most often the anterolateral aspect of the thing, the upper-outer quadrant of the gluteal region, and the mid-deltoid region. Of these three traditional IM sites the **mid-deltoid region** provides the most rapid uptake of most medications as a result of greater tissue perfusion and is therefore the **site of choice**.

Emergency medications can be injected into the body of the tongue or into the sublingual region with every expectation of a more rapid uptake and onset of clinical action. The drug may be administered under the tongue either intra orally or extra orally. Onset of actions approximately 5-10 minutes, if there is effective circulation. However the steps of basic life support must be continued as need while the emergency team awaits the onset of the drugs action

We should remember that the absence of effective circulation neither intravenously nor intramuscularly administered drugs will be effective. Int his situation implementation of ABC's of basic life support rather than drugs should take precedence.

All the injectable emergency drugs are available in the form known as a "Unit dose" or "therapeutic dose".

The 1 ml form of the drug is its adult and not pediatric therapeutic dose. A milliliter is a unit of volume, not of a drug's strength. Administration of the 1 mil form of any emergency drug to an adult victim would be appropriate.

One major exception is Epinephrine. Although the 1 ml form of 1:1000 epinephrine is considered the adult therapeutic dose, a smaller dose 0.3 to 0.5 ml is initially administered, with subsequent doses based on the patient response. Pediatric doses are of necessity proportionately smaller, usually one quarter to one half the adult dose.

The only basic drug that should be available in a preloaded form is epinephrine because in the acute alleric reaction, this drug should be administered as soon is possible.

ACLS drugs are available in preloaded form and are kept separate from basic emergency drugs.

PRIMARY INJECTABLE DRUGS

1.   Drug for acute allergic reaction: Epinephrine (Adrenalin) is the drug of choice for the management of the acute allergic reaction. (Signs and symptoms appearing within 1 hour of drug administration).

Epinephrine is of primary value in the management of the respiratory and cardiovascular manifestations of allergic reactions.

Desirable properties include-

- Rapid onset of action.
- Potent action as a bronchial smooth muscle dilator4 (beta properties).
- Antihistaminic properties.
- Vasopressor properties
- It action on the heart which include.

Increased heart rate, increased systolic blood pressure, decreased diastolic blood pressure, increased cardiac output and increased coronary blood flow.

However undesirable actions include tendency to predispose the heart to arrhythmias and short duration of action.

Therapeutic Indications: Acute allergic reactions, acute asthmatic attacks, cardiac arrest.

Side Effects, Contraindications and Precautions:

- ❖ Tachyarrhythmias may develop.
- ❖ It should be used with caution in pregnancy because it decreases placental blood flow and may induce premature labor.
- ❖ When used all vital signs should be frequently monitored.

Suggested for emergency kit: 1. One reloaded syringe and 3-4 ampoules of 1:1000 epinephrine also available as 1 mg diluted in 10 mil fluid for intravenous administration (1:10,000)

Dosage:

0.01 mg/kg (0.1 ml/kg of 1:10,000 IV), (0.01 ml/kg of 1:1000 IM); may need to repeat after 5 to 10 minutes as needed. Single pediatric doses should not exceed 0.3 mg. Administration of the agent is either subcutaneous or intramuscular/ intralingual.

2.   **Antihistamine**: Drug of choice of <u>Chlorpheniramine</u>. Alternative drug is Diphenhydramine HCL. Antihistamines are given is treatment of the delayed allergic response (onset of symptoms more than 1 hour after administration of the allergen) and in the definitive management of the acute allergic reaction (administered after epinephrine has terminated the acute life threatening phase of the reaction).

Antihistamines are competitive antagonists of histamine. They are more potent in preventing the actions of histamine than in reversing these actions once they develop.

Chlorpheniramine is the choice of an anti histamine as most dental patients are ambulatory and may leave the dental office unescorted. A potential side-effect of many antihistamines is a degree of cortical depression (sedation) that will prevent the patient from leaving the dental office unescorted.

Therapeutic Indications: Delayed allergy, definitive management of acute allergy for local anesthesia, when history of alleged allergy is present.

Side Effects, Contraindications and Precautions:

- Side effects include CNS depression decreased blood pressure and a thicknening of bronchial secretions resulting from the drugs drying action.

56

- Antihitamines are contraindicated in the management of acute asthmatic episodes.

Suggested for emergency kit: Chlorpheniramine 10 mg/ml or Diphen hydramine, 50 mg/ml.

Dosage: Diphenhydramine (Benadry): 1 to 2 mg/kg. IV or IM.

3.   Anticonvulsant: Drug of choice is Diazepam seizure disorders may occur in the dental office in several circumstances: overdose reactions to local anesthetics, epileptic seizures and febrile convulsions.

Diazepam is the preferred drug because diazepam unlike barbiturates will usually terminate seizure activity without the pronounced depression of the respiratory and cardiovascular systems.

Therapeutic indications: Termination of prolonged seizures local anesthetic seizures hyperventilation syndrome thyroid storm.

Side Effect, Contraindications and Precautions:

The major side effects are respiratory depression or arrest. However with careful titration during administration this is unlikely to occur. Sedation can also occur.

Suggested for emergency kig: One 10 ml. vial of diazepam,5 mg/ml.

Dosage:

<5 years:03 mg/kg. with initial dose not exceeding 0.25 mg/kg to a maximum of 0.75 mg/kg total dose for episode, slow IV (or deep IM); maximal total dose, 5 mg; >5 years: 1 mg/dose, slow IV; maximal total dose, 10 mg

4.   Narcotic antagonist: Drug of choice is Naloxone and alternative drug is Nalbuphine. If a narcotic analgesic or pentazocine is included in the drug emergency kit or used for psychosedation techniques a narcotic antagonist must be readily available. Narcotic antagonists are indicated for reversal of narcotic depression including respiratory depression.

Therapeutic Indication: Respiratory depression caused by narcotics or pentazocine.

Side Effects, Contraindications and Precautions: naloxone has been notably free of adverse side effects.

Dosage:

0.01 mg/kg,IV or IM; may repeat with a subsequent dose of 0.1 mg/kg if need.

NOTE:

The duration of nalxone is short shorter than that of the narcotic it is reversing this situation may lead of the narcotic it is reversing. The situation may lead to a recurrence of respiratory depression following a period of apparent recovery. For this reason all patients receiving naloxone must be abserved for at least 1 hour after its administration. Longer acting narcotic antagonist naltrexone should be available in the near future.

Suggested for emergency kit: Naloxone, 0.4 mg/ml (two to three 1 ml ampoules)

SECONDARY INJECTABLE DRUGS:

They are agents that are deemed important but not absolutely essential to the successful management of emergency situations. Their inclusion in the kit is recommended only if the doctor has the background and ability to safely and effectively employ these agents clinically.

1. **Analgesic drug**: Drug of choice is <u>Morphine sulfate</u>. Analgesic medication will be useful during emergency situations in which acute pain or anxiety is present. Pain or anxiety causes an increase in the workload of heart that proves to be detrimental.

    Two such circumstances are acute myocardial infarction and congestive heart failure. The choice of analgesic drug included the narcotic agonists morphine sulphate and meperidine.

2. **Vasopressors**: Drug of choice is <u>Methoxamine</u> and alternative drug is pheylephrine. As epinephrine elicits an extreme anti hypotensive response it is not used in most emergency situations in which a vasopressor is indicated in the dental office.

    It is desirable to utilize a vasopressor that produces a moderate increase in blood pressure without simulating the myocardium. Vasopressors which as Methoxamine and Phenylephrine are drugs producing moderate B.P. elevations through the mechanism of peripheral vasoconstriction.

    Dosage: Methoxamine (Vasoxyl): 0.25 mg/kg, IM ,or 0.08 mg/kg, slow IV.
    Ephedrine: 05 mg/kg IV or IM.

3. **Corticosteroids**: Drug of choice is hydrocortisone sodium succinate and alterative drug is methyl prednisolone sodium succinate.

    Corticosteroids will be employed in the management of the acute allergic reaction only after the acute phase has been brought under control using epinephrine and the antihistamines its primary value is in the prevention of recurrent episode of anaphylaxis and also in the management of acute adrenal insufficiency. Dexamethasone and methylprednisolone, sodium succinate are contraindicate for use in acute adrenal insufficiency.

4. **Antihypoglycemics**: Drug of choice is <u>50% Dextrose solution</u> and alternate drug is Glucagon. It the management of hypoglycemic patient the mode of therapy depends on the patient the mode of therapy depends on the patient's level of consciousness. Oral carbohydrate is the preferred mode of therapy, but if the patient is unconscious oral route must not be employed. Then 50 ml of 50% dextrose solution may be administered intravenously. When the IV (intravenous) route is not available Glucagon may be administered IM (intramuscular).

Dosage:

1. 50% Dextrose: 0.5 to 1 g/kg (1 to 2 ml/kg), IV, until patient regains consciousness.

2. **Glucagon**: 0.5 to 1 mg IM (0.025 to 0.1 mg/kg), may repeat dosing after 20 minutes if need. Maximal single dose is 1 mg.

INJECTABLE DRUGS FOR ACLS

The following drugs are classified as essential drugs in emergency cardiac care by the AHA (American Heart Association). Their use is limited to persons trained in advanced cardiac life support including certain physicians, nurses dental practitioners and some emergency medical technicians.

1. Atropine sulphate:

Use: Management of bradycardia

Action: Atropine is a parasympathetic (vagal) blocking agent; therefore, it increases the patient's heart rate

Dosage : 0.01 mg/kg,IV or IM. For ACLS, 0.02 mg/kg,IV or IM

Side effects: Tachycardia, arrhythmia, dry mouth.

2.   Sodium Bicarbonate ($NaHCO_3$)

Use: Acidosis, Cardiac arrest.

Action: Raises blood pH directly.

Dosage: 1 mEq/kg, slow IV at 10 minute intervals, as needed during resuscitation.

Side effects: Alkalosis, hypernatremia.

3.   Calcium Chloride:

Use: Asystole, hypotension, electromechanical dissociation.

Action: Increased cardiac contractility.

Dosage: 0.2 ml/kg of 10% calcium chloride IV willprovide 20 mg/kg, every 10 minutes as needed.

Side effects: Phlebitis

4.   Lidocaine:

Use: Lidocaine is used to manage ventricular arrhythmias (ventricular extrasystoles and ventricular tachycardia).

Note: Only "cardiac lidocaine" may be used for this purpose. Dental lidocaine should not be injected intravenously.

Action: Lidocaine depresses automaticity and suppresses ectopic ventricular pacemakers.

Dosage: 1 mg/kg, IV

Side effects: Sedation, local anesthetic toxicity in high doses (seizures)

PRIMARY NON-INJECTABLE DRUGS

1. **Oxygen**: The most important drug in the entire emergency kit is oxygen. E cylinder is the minimal acceptable size as it provides oxygen for approx 30 minutes because emergencies occur in other parts of the dental office than the dental chair, oxygen must be available anywhere within the office.

2. **Vasodilator:** Drug of choice is Nitroglycerin and alternative drug is Amyl nitrite. They are used in the immediate management of chest pain (angina pectoris, acute myocardial infarction).

SECONDARY NON-INJECTABLE DRUGS

1. **Respiratory Stimulant:** Drug of choice is aromatic Ammonia. It is available in a silver gray vaporole, which is crushed and placed under the victim's nose until respiratory stimulation is affected. Aromatic ammonia acts by irritating the mucous membrane of the upper respiratory tract, thereby stimulating the respiratory and vasomotor centers of the medulla, thus in turn increases respiration and blood pressure.

NOTE: Ammonia is used with caution in persons with COPD or asthma as it precipitates bronchospasm.

2. **Antihypoglycemic (oral)**: Agent of choice is the Carbohydrate. Antihypoglycemic agents are useful in the management of hypoglycemic

reactions occurring in patients with hypoglycemia. A chocolate candy or hard candy should be available in the dental office for use in the conscious patient with hypoglycemia.

3. **Bronchodilating agent**: Drug of choice is <u>Metaproterenol</u>. Alternative drugs are Epinephrine and Isoproterenol. Asthmatic patients and patients with allergic reactions manifested primarily by respiratory difficulty will require the use of bronchodilator drugs. One inhaler of Metaproterenol is suggested for the emergency kit.

MEDICOLEGAL CONSIDERATIONS

Recently, much ha been written about the legal implications of practicing dentistry because each year many dentists are used.

Most claims and law suits are brought aginst dentists because of an allegedly undesired result arising from desired treatment. Complaints of physical damage to components of the mouth are frequent, particularly nerve damage resulting in temporary or permanent loss of sensation and/or loss of control of portions of the mouth.

Although malpractice complaints because of medical emergencies in dental offices constitute a minority of the total number of lawsuits against dentists, the life and death nature of medical emergencies makes these cases among he most serious in terms of potential injury to the patient and of the dentists liability.

Lawsuits for damages because of temporary paresthesia, a broken needle or permanent cosmetic injuries pale in comparison to lawsuits brought because of brain damage or death from improperly administered CPR during a cardiac arrest emergency6. Lawsuits resulting from medical emergencies are based on injuries and medical consequences to the patient that demand the highest jury verdicts and the highest defense cost.

Therefore it is appropriate and timely to consider low dentists can avoid being used, and if they are sued, what it will take to win.

Several forms are commonly used which include ADA-recommended medical history questionnaire and USE medical history questionnaire. They represent forms that have been accepted throughout the profession and can be important evidence for the dentist in a lawsuit brought by a Patient.

THE JURY SYSTEM

Unless a dentist has agreed with a patient before hand to resolve a dispute in any way other than the judicial system, such as through arbitration, the existing judicial system in each community and state is the mechanism through which a complaint of malpractice will be resolved. More particularly, if a medical emergency has arisen in a dental office and the patient claims to have been injured because of negligence during the medical emergency, and subsequently files a lawsuit, the case will be disposed of ultimately at trial by the jury

CONCLUSION

Although pediatric medical emergencies are rare in a dental office, when it does occur, it should be managed with definitive treatment plan. Early recognition of the problem is required to prevent dire consequences. Physically and physiologically immature pediatric patients require efficient and timely treatment in case of medical emergency.

Successful management of medical emergencies requires preparation, prevention and knowledge of definitive management not only by the dentist but also by the supporting dental staff members.

For all emergencies:
1. Discontinue dental treatment
4. Monitor vital signs
2. Call for assistance; activate in-office oxygen and emergency kit
5. If trained in support procedures, provide emergency support
3. Position patient comfortably and monitor airway
6. Activate CPR and call for emergency medical services

Condition	Signs and symptoms	Treatment	Drug dosage	Drug delivery*
Allergic reaction (mild or delayed)	Hives; itching; edema; erythema; skin; mucosa congestion	1. Discontinue all sources of allergy causing substances 2. Administer diphenhydramine	Diphenhydramine 1 mg/kg Child: 10-25 mg qid Adult: 25-50 mg qid	Oral
Allergic reaction (sudden onset): anaphylaxis	Urticaria; itching; flushing; hives; rhinitis; wheezing/difficulty breathing; bronchospasm; laryngeal edema; weak pulse; marked fall in blood pressure; loss of consciousness	This is a true life-threatening emergency 1. Call for emergency medical services 2. Administer epinephrine 3. Administer oxygen 4. Monitor vital signs 5. Transport to emergency medical facility by advanced medical responders	Epinephrine 1:1000 0.01 mg/kg every 5 min until recovery or until help arrives	IM or SubQ
Acute asthmatic attack	Shortness of breath; wheezing; coughing; tightness in chest; cyanosis; tachycardia	1. Sit patient upright or in a comfortable position 2. Administer oxygen 3. Administer bronchodilator 4. If bronchodilator is ineffective, administer epinephrine 5. Call for emergency medical services with transportation for advanced care if indicated	1. Albuterol (patient's or emergency kit inhaler) 2. Epinephrine 1:1000 0.01 mg/kg every 15 min as needed	Inhale IM or SubQ
Local anesthetic toxicity	Light-headedness; changes in vision and/or speech; metallic taste; changes in mental status; confusion; agitation; tinnitus; tremor; seizure; tachypnea; bradycardia; unconsciousness; cardiac arrest	1. Assess and support airway, breathing, and circulation (CPR if warranted) 2. Administer oxygen 3. Monitor vital signs 4. Call for emergency medical services with transportation for advanced care if indicated	Supplemental oxygen	Mask
Local anesthetic reaction: vasoconstrictor	Anxiety; tachycardia/ palpitations; restlessness; headache; tachypnea; chest pain; cardiac arrest	1. Reassure patient 2. Assess and support airway, breathing, and circulation (CPR if warranted) 3. Administer oxygen 4. Monitor vital signs 5. Call for emergency medical services with transportation for advanced care if indicated	Supplemental oxygen	Mask
Overdose: benzodiazepine	Somnolence; confusion; diminished reflexes; respiratory depression; apnea; respiratory arrest; cardiac arrest	1. Assess and support airway, breathing, and circulation (CPR if warranted) 2. Administer oxygen 3. Monitor vital signs 4. If severe respiratory depression, establish IV access and reverse with flumazenil 5. Monitor recovery (for at least 2 hours after the last dose of flumazenil) and call for emergency medical services with transportation for advanced care if indicated	Flumazenil 0.01-0.02 mg/kg (maximum: 0.2 mg); may repeat at 1 min intervals not to exceed a cumulative dose of 0.05 mg/kg or 1 mg, whichever is lower	IV (if IV access is not available, may be given IM)

For all emergencies
1. Discontinue dental treatment
2. Call for assistance/someone to bring oxygen and emergency kit
3. Position patient, ensure open and unobstructed airway
4. Monitor vital signs
5. Be prepared to support respiration, support circulation, provide cardiopulmonary resuscitation (CPR), and call for emergency medical services

Condition	Signs and symptoms	Treatment	Drug dosage	Drug delivery*
Overdose: narcotic	Decreased responsiveness; respiratory depression; respiratory arrest; cardiac arrest	1. Assess and support airway, breathing, and circulation (CPR if warranted) 2. Administer oxygen 3. Monitor vital signs 4. If severe respiratory depression, reverse with naxolone 5. Monitor recovery (for at least 2 hours after the last dose of naxolone) and call for emergency medical services with transportation for advanced care if indicated	Naxolone 0.1 mg/kg up to 2 mg. May be repeated to maintain reversal.	IV, IM, or SubQ
Seizure	Warning aura-disorientation, blinking, or blank stare; uncontrolled muscle movements; muscle rigidity; unconsciousness; postictal phase-sleepiness, confusion, amnesia, slow recovery	1. Recline and position to prevent injury 2. Ensure open airway and adequate ventilation 3. Monitor vital signs 4. If status is epilepticus, give diazepam and call for emergency medical services with transportation for advanced care if indicated	Diazepam Child up to 5 yrs: 0.2-0.5 mg slowly every 2-5 min with maximum-5 mg Child 5 yrs and up: 1 mg every 2-5 min with maximum-10 mg	IV
Syncope (fainting)	Feeling of warmth; skin pale and moist; pulse rapid initially then gets slow and weak; dizziness; hypotension; cold extremities; unconsciousness	1. Recline, feet up 2. Loosen clothing that may be binding 3. Ammonia inhales 4. Administer oxygen 5. Cold towel on back of neck 6. Monitor recovery	Ammonia in vials	Inhale

*Legend: IM = intramuscular   IV = intravenous   SubQ = subcutaneous

BIBLIOGRAPHY

1. **Morrow G.T.:** Designing a drug kit, Dent Clin North Am 26(1):21-33, 1982

2. Malamed SF: Managing medical emergencies. J Am Dent Assoc 124:40-53, 1993.

3. **McCarthy EM**: Sudden, unexpected dental office. J Am Dent Assoc 83:1091, 1971

4. **Goldberger E:** Treatment of cardiac emergencies, ed 5, St. Louis, 1990, Mosby.

5. **Goodsen JM, Moore PA:** Life-threatening reactions after pedodontic sedation: an assessment of opioid, local anesthetic, and antiemetic drug interaction. J Am Dent Assoc 107:239, 1983

6. **McCarthy FM:** Emergencies in dental practice, ed 3, Philadeplphia, 1979, WB Saunder.

7. **Rossen R, Kabat H, Anderson JP:** Acute arrest of the cerebral circulationin man. Arch Neurol Psychiatr 50:510, 1943

8. **Malamed SF**: Beyond the basics: emergency medicine in dentistry. A Am Dent Assoc 128(7):843-854, 1997

9. **Little JW and Falce DA:** Dental management of the medically compromised patient. Ed 5, St. Louis, 1997 Mosby.

10. **Goldberger** E: Treatment of cardiac emergencies, ed 5, St Louis, 1990, Mosby

11. **Hegenbarth MA**, Committee on Drugs. Preparing for Pediatric Emergencies: Drugs to Consider, American Academy of Pediatrics. Pediatrics 2008;121(2);433-43.

12. **Pediatric Advanced Life Support**: 2010 American Heart Association Guidelines for Cardiopulmonary Resuscitation and Emergency Cardio-vascular Care. Circulation 2010;122;S876-S908.

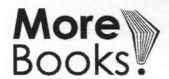

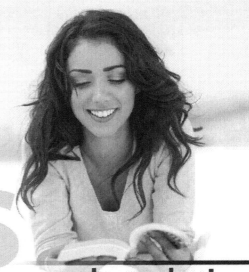

yes

i want morebooks!

Buy your books fast and straightforward online - at one of the world's fastest growing online book stores! Environmentally sound due to Print-on-Demand technologies.

Buy your books online at

www.get-morebooks.com

Kaufen Sie Ihre Bücher schnell und unkompliziert online – auf einer der am schnellsten wachsenden Buchhandelsplattformen weltweit!
Dank Print-On-Demand umwelt- und ressourcenschonend produziert.

Bücher schneller online kaufen

www.morebooks.de

OmniScriptum Marketing DEU GmbH
Heinrich-Böcking-Str. 6-8
D - 66121 Saarbrücken
Telefax: +49 681 93 81 567-9

info@omniscriptum.de
www.omniscriptum.de

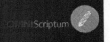

30354066R00047

Made in the USA
San Bernardino, CA
11 February 2016